BONNIE'S THEORY

FINDING

THE RIGHT EXERCISE

BONNIE FRANKEL

And

Linda C. Furlong

Library of Congress Cataloging-in-Publication data
Names: Frankel, Bonnie, author. | Furlong, Linda C., author
Title: **Bonnie's Theory**: Finding the right Exercise
     Bonnie Frankel; and Linda C. Furlong
Description: San Bernardino, CA: Kindle; Ingram Sparks,
[2019] | Summary: The elements of Fire, Air, Earth and
Water have been used throughout the centuries for health
and fitness. This book introduces a unique theory of finding
the right exercise by identifying with your personal type.
Once you find your element type you'll stick with exercising
and maintaining fitness for the rest of your life.—Publisher.
Identifiers: ISBN: 9781979966771
Subjects: LCSH: Frankel, Bonnie. | Exercise—
Psychological aspects. | Exercise—Health aspects. |
Health. | Four elements (Philosophy) | Typology
(Psychology) | Four temperaments. | Breast—Cancer—
Patients—United States—Biography. | Divorced women—
United States--Biography. | Women runners—Biography. |
Self-actualization (Psychology) in middle age.
Classification: LCC: GV481.2 .F73 2019 | DDC: 613.7/1—
dc23

Copyright © August 05, 2019 Bonnie
Frankel   All   rights   reserved
The characters and events portrayed in this
book are fictitious. Any similarity to real
persons, living or dead, is coincidental and
not   intended   by   the   author.
No part of this book may be reproduced, or
stored in a retrieval system, or transmitted
in any form or by any means, electronic,
mechanical, photocopying, recording, or
otherwise,   without   express   written
permission of the publisher.

All rights reserved.

ISBN-13: 9781979966771
ISBN-10: 9781996677X

ACKNOWLEDGEMENT

With my sincere gratitude to my dearest friend, Mary Beyer, for always giving me her love and unconditional support.

BONNIE FRANKEL

"A healthy body means a healthy mind. Get your heart rate up and you get the blood flowing through your body to your brain; look at Albert Einstein. He rode a bicycle. He was also an early student of Jazzercise. You never saw Einstein lift his shirt, but he had a six pack under there," Steve Carrell[1]

---

[1] https://www.brainyquote.com/authors/steve_carell

BONNIE FRANKEL

INTRODUCTION

"You want me to do something. Tell me I can't do it." Maya Angelou [2]

Take control of your life and seize the vitality you were meant to enjoy. This is something I know you can do by choosing the right exercise.

By sharing my theory, I'm going to show you how to accomplish the fitness results you've always dreamed. You'll learn the secret to enjoying an exercise that's right up-

---

[2] https://azquotes.com/quote/52890

your-alley. Not only will you become physically, emotionally and mentally fit, it will enable you to live in a sweeter place within your soul.

I decided to write this book because many people ask me what my secret is to fitness. The simple answer is when you find the right exercise it's like finding your BFF. The right exercise will make the difference between you being active and fit or, just being an unfit couch potato.

Do you find yourself avoiding exercise? Do you joke by telling others that you're allergic to it? Do you say things like the following anonymous quote?

"I exercised once but found out I was allergic to it. My skin flushed, and my heart raced. I got sweaty and short of breath...." Minion quote [3]

Do you avoid exercise because you think it will deplete your energy to do other tasks? There are those people that think this way.

President Donald Trump's view on exercise is that the human body is like a battery with a finite amount of energy that exercise depletes. Experts say this argument is flawed because the human body becomes

---

[3]https://onsizzle.com/i/i-exercised-once-but-found-out-i-was-allergic-to-e753c2a4b63a41fba16b319277e02314

stronger with exercise.

In contrast to how President Trump feels, George W. Bush plays golf and rides a mountain bike. He feels it's important to stay healthy by continued exercise.

Everyone has a different response to exercise. The most important thing is that you enjoy it so you'll continue doing it. When you exercise, only you know what it feels like.

Throughout my life I've heard many fitness specialists promising that "their" program is the only one that will make you lean and mean in record-breaking time. I get furious because it's just not true.

"The fitness industry has long thrived off the well-intended coming through their doors and signing up with dreams of self-improvement, only to fade into their couches. Those who stick with it often feel like hamsters on tread mills." Mary Pilon [4]

Promises like these are hard to keep. Every one of us is different and your exercises should be different as well. Fitness is a process, not a quick fix.

Kate Hudson likes the saying

---

[4] https://www.brainyquote.com/quotes/mary_pilon_900755

that if you motivate the mind the body will follow. That it is a slow process, so don't make it slower by quitting.

Finding the right exercise is going to challenge and change the way you view exercise. It will become an acquired habit that you will look forward to doing.

Under your personal element, you'll find the correct exercise that matches your psychological makeup. It will make your exercise more enjoyable and less of a chore; thus, creating the ability to stay on track and maintain fitness for life.

"The right exercise puts you

in the right frame of mind to become a more fit you." Bonnie Frankel.

Before we begin looking for your personal element, let me take you back to where it all began. I feel by sharing how I found the right exercise that changed my life, will also inspire you to change yours.

TRANSITION

I grew up in the Bel-Air area in Southern California living a privileged life style among the rich and famous.

My parents were strong advocates of exercise and education, and always encouraged me to work if I wasn't enrolled in some form of education.

At one of my jobs, I worked for the late Jay Sebring as his personal secretary and office manager for Sebring Inc. As his company grew, he needed me to help with hair cutting demonstrations at high-end department stores. This inspired me to get my barber's license. Unfortunately, in the middle of my training, he was killed along with Sharon Tate and others in the gruesome Manson Murders. In spite of this tragedy, I continued to finish barber school and got my license to cut hair. I found a space at the Burbank Studios to open my own hairstyling salon. This is where I met my husband.

After three years of dating we married, and I continued to live an affluent life style. We enjoyed having two homes, drove fashionable cars, and belonged to a country club where we were avid tennis players. I also had housekeepers that helped me juggle my commitments. We traveled a lot and attended many charitable tennis events.

Six months into my marriage, disease unexpectedly invaded my life. I was diagnosed with breast cancer and endured many surgeries. As if the process of cancer wasn't challenging enough, I discovered my husband was having an affair with a close friend of ours. We tried counseling, but it failed. Divorce was in the works.

At this time, I decided to close my salon and created a bucket list including: yoga, gymnastics, scuba diving, skeet shooting, hiking, water skiing, art school, classical piano lessons, continuing tennis, and swimming. Little did I know at the time, the bucket list helped me to rehabilitate as the process of healing, fitness, and change began.

"In terms of fitness, and battling through cancer, exercise helps you stay strong physically and mentally," Greta Waltz[5]

I became unfulfilled with my role as being Mrs. Doctor Frankel and developed an insatiable yearn

---

[5]https://www.allinspiration.com/a/cancer-quotes-and-sayings/4/

to find my own identity. Unexpectedly, the process of divorcing made my life so intolerable, I stopped exercising and became emotionally unstable. Doom and gloom set in, as the stress of divorcing turned out to be more than I could cope with. I felt like a failure.

Feelings of despair clouded my thinking, and depression affected my better judgment. So, following in my mother's and my best friend's footsteps, I tried to commit suicide. I even failed at that.

It took time for me to forgive myself, but I innately returned to exercise. Since exercising helped me through my bout with cancer, I felt it would help me to recover from the trauma of divorcing.

"For me, exercise is more than just physical – it's therapeutic." Michelle Obama.[6]

When the process of my divorce was finally completed, the judge gave me a simple piece of advice, "Go back to college and find out what you want to do with your life."

---

[6]http://healthawaredot.com.wordpress.com/2019/12for-me-exercise-is-more-than-just-physical-michelle-obama/6/

I thought "OMG! Is he out of his mind?", but took up the challenge anyway, and went back to college at the ripe age of forty-four. Lucky for me it was a trend that older women were following. This way I wouldn't stand out like a sore thumb, so I thought.

"The choices you make in life make you." John wooden [7]

At nineteen, I had dropped out of college due to learning disabilities, and now I was back at the same school with a younger

---

[7]https:// www.azquotes.com/quote/549720

generation. I felt like a misfit adjusting to a different life style; no maids, no glamour, no rich and famous.

Most of my classes were filled with students young enough to be my kids. Where were the older women? This experience was intimidating causing a lot of anxiety, and a fear of failing again. What I didn't know was that I had a great surprise ahead of me.

FINDING MY RIGHT EXERCISE

One of my young school pals suggested we take a running class. I thought why not? Without knowing it, my theory was about to begin. This class was the golden key to a new me, and I began to weave a new segment of my life.

I was astonished to find that running was the exercise that lit up my life, and still does. Even though I had done different types of exercises in the past, none of them held a candle to my new-found passion. I was hooked and didn't know why.

"I've always loved running…it is something you could do by yourself under your own power. You can go in any direction, fast or slow as you wanted, fighting the wind if you feel like it, seeking out new sights, just on the strength of your feet and the courage of your lungs," Jesse Owens.[8]

While enjoying my new-found love of running, I began noticing other joyous changes in my life. As I trained, I became more physically and psychologically fit than I had

---

[8] https://feelthewindandjoy.wordpress.com/

ever been before.

Prior to running, my school chums gave me the nick-name of "Bonster the Monster". I was difficult to deal with and had a "princess" mentality. My attitude was negative, and I complained all the time.

"Movement is a medicine for creating change in a person's physical, emotional, and mental states." Carol Welch[9]

The anxiety I had while trying to cover up my learning disabilities caused me to develop a superiority complex thinking it would make

---

[9]https://www.pinterest.com/micristopuede/movement-is-a-medicine-for-creating-change-in-a-pe/

me feel more confident. Instead I felt isolated. Concentrating at lectures was difficult for me, so I carried a tape recorder. This allowed me to later listen to the lectures over, and over again. It was time consuming and a drag! After a few weeks of running, I felt more alert and relied less and less on my tape recordings. My retention of the lecture information was improving, and I was finally able to dump the recorder. Halleluiah!

My relationships with others improved, and I developed a healthier and more positive attitude.

"Exercise and application produce order in our affairs,

health of body, cheerfulness of mind, and these make us precious to our friends." Thomas Jefferson.[10]

Since I got rid of the chip on my shoulder, the kids changed my name from "Bonster the Monster", to "Energizer Bunny". I started to feel more connected with the college scene, and myself. No longer did I feel superior but felt more integrated and comfortable with my surroundings.

"I've learned that even when I have pains, I don't have to be

---

[10] https://www.azquotes.com/quote/522958

one." Maya Angelou [11]

The feelings and results running gave me were extraordinary. It honed, toned and reshaped my body and mind like no other exercise I had done before. The more miles I ran, the younger I felt. I was addicted.

One day I asked my coach why this was, and he just smiled. He replied with this answer, "Isn't that something, and as long as you can put on a pair of shoes, you'll keep on running," and he was as right as rain.

---

[11] https://www.goodreads.com/quotes/40498-i-ve-learned-that-even-when-i-have-pains-i-don-t

CHANGING A RULE

After taking the running class, the track coach asked me to join the women's track team. I gladly accepted this challenge and became a competitor representing Santa Monica College.

My dad attended one of my races and was yelling, "Bonnie you're going to have a heart attack!" just as I beat a younger athlete by a hair. It truly was a kodak moment for the both of us as he was soon to be diagnosed with Alzheimer Disease.

The common belief that you get feeble when you get older, didn't apply to me. It was quite the contrary. I felt stronger. My physical strength was equal with runners that were half my age, and it also ignited my competitive spirit.

Finding the right exercise helped new successes to open up. After attending Santa Monica College, the second time around, I graduated with honors in track, high academic grades and an AA degree. This allowed me to advance my education by transferring to a four-year university.

In hopes of obtaining a Bachelor of Arts Degree, I transferred to Loyola Marymount

University in Westchester, California. It had smaller classes which would help me with my learning disabilities. Since running played such a crucial role with creating the new me, joining the cross-country team was a major priority. I met with the head coach, and he told me that due to the current N.C.A.A., (National Collegiate Athletics Association) rule, my eligibility time limit to run cross-country had expired. Loyola is considered a Division One Collegiate Institute. At this college level, the N.C.A.A., had a Five-Year Rule stating; once a student started college, and wanted to compete at a Division One level, they only had five years to do it.

When I had initially enrolled at Santa Monica College in 1962 at the age of seventeen, my time clock started ticking. My five years was up in 1967.

This rule made me furious because it not only affected me but also affected other women in the same predicament. The honor and privilege of competing in Division One collegiate sports would not be available to us. It was unjust, and I didn't see why it couldn't be changed because the N.C.A.A. didn't even govern women's sports until 1982. So, I began the process of fighting this rule.

"If you don't like something, change it. If you can't change it, change your attitude." Maya Angelou[12]

The powerful media, not the fake media, as it is referred to today, caught wind of my plight. They were supportive in helping me challenge this rule by giving me full-blown national coverage. It allowed me to eventually win my battle.

They said things like, "In her most recent incarnation, Bonnie

---

[12] https://www.brainyquote.com/quotes/maya_angelou_1

has turned athletics on its ear and in doing so she's forcing women everywhere to reconsider their own physical potential."

While I was waiting for the decision on the rule change, I trained with an Olympic running coach. She added swimming and running in the water to my training regimen.

This enabled me to maintain the new self I was experiencing. It also showed me another way to run distance and sprint by using the natural resistance of water. This provided me with an alternative way to exercise without risking injury.

During this time, I continued my fight against the N.C.A.A., and after a lot of hard work, my goal of changing the five-year rule was actualized. It was nicknamed the "Bonnie Rule". This rule would allow women that had entered college before 1982 to compete in a Division One Collegiate Sport.

"Always go with passions, never ask yourself if it's realistic or not." Deepak Chopra[13]

The media commented that with every stride, I was changing

---

[13] https://www.brainyquote.com/quotes/deepak_chopra_453997

history. Unfortunately, by the time the rule was changed, the cross-country season was over.

Lucky for me the head coach of the women's swim team at Loyola had seen me training in the water and was impressed with my speed. He asked me if I'd like the opportunity to join the team. I was so honored and grateful to take advantage of the newly changed rule; I happily accepted the challenge. This allowed me to rekindle my love of competing with college kids. They were talented and always full of fresh energy.

Under the rule change, I made history by becoming the oldest woman to compete in a Division One Collegiate Sport. I was proud to represent the baby boomer generation. We were now able to compete with the younger Generation X, also known as the Baby Busts.

HOW MY THEORY BEGAN

When I graduated from Loyola, the Head coach at Santa Monica High School asked me to train with the track and cross-country teams. He saw this as an opportunity for me to inspire his students. I happily accepted this invitation of leadership as I would be inspiring these highs school kids as well as experiencing their glorious energy. The coach would tease them by saying, "Are you going to let this old lady beat you?" Sometimes I would run against the football team with the coaches taking bets as to which one of us would win. This relationship grew into me becoming one of the assistant coaches for the teams.

This same coach could see that, although I was helping train his student athletes, and running with them as well, it wasn't challenging my own abilities. It turned out I was faster than the girls on the team, and some of the boys. I told him about my goal of trying to qualify for the Olympic Trials, so he invited me to train with the Santa Monica Track Club. This was a group of elite athletes. Some of them were being coached for the Olympics, and some of them did it for the sheer pleasure.

Running at this level of expertise improved my running times. I was becoming a world-class runner by competing in open races, and in the national and world-class Masters' competitions that are age-graded.

I was in better shape than I had ever been and was convinced that when a person found the right exercise, as I did, it would do the same for them. In the back of my mind I kept wondering why the athletes I was coaching, were drawn to a specific exercise and how would they know it was the right one for them?

I began looking at the kids

through a different set of eyes as they trained and raced. There were a few of them that just weren't connecting with their choice of exercise and yet there were others that were.

Loaded with curiosity, I decided to go to the library to see if I could find an answer. The places I visited had oodles of information about different cultures and their theories on the subject.

As, I focused on why people are drawn to certain types of exercises, the result became crystal clear. There was an idea flowing through the pieces of information that connected to the four elements of nature; Fire, Air, Earth, and Water. These elements have a big influence over our psychological make up and why we do the things we do.

It had always been in the forefront of my mind that these four elements are basic to all things in life, and each element has explicit characteristics that define our psychological makeup. The descriptive characteristics of each element helped me develop a concrete theory. While I carefully read the information about these elements, it just re-enforced their validity and my connection to them.

Seeing the world in terms of the four elements is a tradition that dates back many years. History accepted that these elements made up all matter and are the cornerstones of science, medicine and philosophy as we know it today.[14] In many cultures, the elements represent the basic principles of life, and different systems have delineated them in various ways.[15]

We can learn a lot about a person just by understanding their

---

[14]Learning-center.homesciencetools.com/article/four-elements-science/

[15]https://www.tarot.com/articles/astrology/elements-fire-earth-air-water

elemental make-up. The human temperament is the result of the elements within us. Everyone differs in the way they express each element – whether it's expressed in a clear way, or in a distorted way. [16]

These four elements have existed in western thinking since pre-historic Greece. They can also be found in the Hindu religion, Chinese culture and Native American practices. The ancients had profound insight as they, too, attributed personality and emotional traits to each element. This enabled them to understand

---

[16] https://www.pandoraastrology.com/blog/personality-flawsl-4-elements/

the mind and to manifest the spiritual into reality.

Hippocrates used the four elements, Fire, Air, Earth, and Water, in developing his medical theories. He connected them to the balance and purity of bodily fluids, which are known as Humors; blood, yellow bile, black bile, and phlegm. It was felt that these four bodily fluids affected personality traits and behaviors. This was the medical concept of Humourism.

"If we could give every individual the right amount of nourishment and exercise, not too little and not too much, we

would have found the safest way to health," Hippocrates.[17]

These Humors were also connected to four different types of temperaments; active, sluggish, irritable, and sad. If the bodily fluids were out of balance with each other, it would affect a person's mental and physical well-being.

Hippocrates believed we all have a dominant Humor that reflects specific personality types. It is also true of the four elements.

In modern times, Carl Jung, psychiatrist and founder of

---

[17] brainyquote.com/quotes/hippocrates_153531

Analytical Psychology, looked at Hippocrates' theory of the Humors, and the basic temperaments. He took Hippocrates' temperaments and connected them to the four elements and looked at the ancient astrological zodiac signs. Jung then connected it all to create his own personality theory. This led to the development of the Myers-Briggs Personality Inventory which is widely used and accepted by psychologists and counselors today. Jung credited astrologers for their insight and influence on his work with personality theory.[18]

---

[18]thelivingsky.wordpress.com/2014/10/25/the-personality-18

"I am not what happened to me, I am what I choose to become." Carl Jung[19]

So, if the four elements affect your body and your mind, wouldn't it stand to reason that you should choose the correct physical movement that connects with your personal element? Each of us has sprinklings of all four, but there is only one element that defines us.

Through my search, I found the one element that best described my

---

18theory-of-carl-Jung-and-the-four-distinct-astrological-temperaments/

19https://www.goodreads.com/quotes/50795-i-am-not-what-happened-to-me-i-am-what

nature. It confirmed what I already suspected. I quickly identified with the Fire element - the element that drives my passion.

I do most of my running outdoors. It's as if I was performing a fast dance surrounded by the beauty of nature. The run enhances my mind and allows me to release my emotions through the activity of my body. I feel free, with no boundaries, and it becomes my way of meditating. My run can be done with others or alone, which adheres to my exercise nature.

This discovery took me on an unexpected path in the world of exercise. Finding the right exercise rocked my world and has continued to do so for a lifetime. I thought that if others could find the right exercise that was meant for them, it would surely give them the same effect. I just had to figure out how to share it with those I trained.

My mind began churning, and through this wealth of information my theory started to take shape. My decision was made. I took the four elements, FIRE, AIR, EARTH, and WATER, and identified the following markers for each of them: their individual personality traits, what triggers their emotional re-actions, and their exercise nature. This would dictate what element category a person fell into, and what exercise would be right for them. I wrote down my information in a small booklet and thus the "Bonnie Theory" was born. A theory I was going to use as I later trained my cross-country teams and others.

BUILDING MY CROSS-COUNTRY TEAM

While I was training and coaching at Santa Monica, the athletic director at Loyola called me out of the blue and asked me if I would be interested in taking over the helm as head coach for the cross-country teams. I excitedly accepted his offer, but in order to take the job, I sadly had to leave coaching at Santa Monica High.

The media got wind of the news and printed, "The young men and women who decide to run cross-country at Loyola are in for a unique experience. Bonnie is a free-spirited new age thinker who basks in her individuality. She hopes to use her enthusiasm to educate others to the glory of movement at any age."

In my first head coaching job at Loyola, I was one of the few women head coaches that coached both men and women teams at the NCAA Division One level. I was honored by being part of the chosen few. The Athletic Director's goal was for me to improve the team's reputation in our West Coast Conference.

Student athletes didn't want to

be on the cross-country team because the program had a bad history. The athletes had no respect for some of the previous coaches, the program was poorly run, and the team always came in last place. The upside to my hire was that I loved the challenge.

My first order of business was to recruit runners, but I only had a small window of time to accomplish this. I spoke at student orientations, recruited by word of mouth, talked to high school coaches, and even asked other Loyola coaches if they had any athletes that would like to cross-train with running. I was also able to offer partial scholarships to entice quality athletes.

At one of the orientations I met darling Keisha, and her family. The school had an athletics booth which attracted her attention. Keisha told me she used to participate in track and field as a sprinter in high school but gave it up in her last season.

We chatted and discussed her joining the women's cross-country team. Keisha shared that she never ran cross-country because long distance terrified her. The possibility of not being number one, like she was in sprinting, got in the way of her ego. Something from her past made her feel if she wasn't perfect at what she did, she wouldn't do it.

Her high school coach told her that if she didn't run cross-country, Keisha wouldn't be able to get stronger or build endurance which would benefit her sprinting. In the realm of a runner's world, it is considered beneficial to run both track and cross-country because they complement one another with endurance, speed and strength. Her personality appeared to be very charismatic, enthusiastic, uplifting, and was laced with an abundance of energy.

Although I felt that she was

concealing something, she wasn't ready to share it with me. Keisha talked a mile a minute, and I envisioned her feet would follow suit due to her "Chatty Kathy" persona.

"Wow!" I thought. Our women's team would have a runner that could inspire them with her magical fast feet. Her body, on the other hand, looked extremely lean; not toned like a sprinter. Sprinters are usually more muscular than distance runners. If she joined the team, maybe we could get some meat on those bones to help with her muscle mass.

As I continued to listen to

Keisha, I observed her with more depth. Behind the shield and spiel was a different type of persona. She was overly obsessive about being perfect, had low self-esteem, and was unusually cautious. This appeared to be indicative of an anorexia nervosa personality disorder which would explain why she was so thin.

For some reason she was punishing her body, but I never really found out what triggered it. Her body was being ravaged by her feelings. Her ego was in full play repeating negative thoughts of: "You'll never be good enough."

*"**What a liberation to realize that the voice in my head is not who I am.**" Eckhart Tolle* [20]

I wondered what I could do to convince her to join the team. Even though she preferred sprinting, I knew she was also capable of challenging the distance run.

*"**You are what you do, not what you say you'll do.**" Carl Jung* [21]

---

[20] https://www.brainyquote.com/quotes/eckhart_tolle_571627

[21] https://www.goodreads.com/quotes/3240-you-are-what-you-do-not-what-you-say-you-ll

I shared my story about how finding my true element helped change me physically, emotionally and mentally. Then I suggested we find out which element she was linked with by looking at my new theory booklet to determine if cross-country running was a good fit for her.

It turned out that she was also a fire element which meant running all distances was a perfect fit. She was excited at this discovery and agreed to give cross-country a chance.

Keisha ran on the balls of her feet, as some sprinters do, so I nicknamed her "Twinkle Toes". I told her not to be concerned with anything, and just enjoy what she liked to do which was simply to run.

I knew that going back to running would help to elucidate her anorexic personality type. Why? Because when you are doing an exercise you love, re-fueling your body becomes a natural and necessary thing to do. It can then perform at its max and fitness returns since your mind and body are living in a healthy union. It's like putting gas in your car to keep it humming and running.

I encouraged her to run more flat-footed for long distances, but more importantly was her passion for the run was in full swing. Finally feeling successful, her negative emotions were dwindling. Her ego was in the present moment, not reliving the past. Keisha was no longer haunted by the feeling of not being good enough. She was able to put on a few pounds and built up her muscle tone.

Keisha was interviewed by the media, and stated, "It's so great having Bonnie as a coach. She runs along with us and never yells when we make mistakes because she knows about the pain we go through."

When I left Loyola, she begged me to stay, but it was time for me to move on. Keisha eventually went on to become team captain of the woman's cross-country team.

As I continued my recruiting to build numbers on my teams, I had to take any student athlete that would be willing to run in order to meet team quotas to race. If not, Loyola would have a major problem, and I would be jobless.

The cross-country team resembled the movie 'The Bad News Bears', so I nick-named them just that. As we began team training in preparation to race, some of them were late to practice looking disheveled. At times they would only wear their high-top tennis shoes, and one girl even came to a race barefoot. They had a sour-grapes disposition and were always complaining about something. I felt that we needed to set standards and expectations.

Since there were no written rules for them to abide by, I created some rules with the help of my team captains. At first, some of the athletes thought they were too rigid but then some of them saw their benefits. When I tried to discipline those that kept breaking the rules, the Loyola athletic department wouldn't back me up. It was very disappointing and frustrating.

Despite the unruliness, it took two seasons for me to bring the team to a respectable place in our West Coast Conference, but we did it. The 'Bad News Bears', was on their journey to transforming into the 'Good News Bears'.

While training them, I mentally placed my teams in two groups. Group one was sportively exercising within their correct element. This group was truly in alignment with their choice of physical exercise. They continuously performed well in their training and racing and were injury free.

Group two appeared to be out of alignment with their exercise of choice. They were performing poorly in their training and racing, and were more prone to injuries. They always looked forlorn.

I needed to see if group two was doing the exercise they were meant to do. The only way I could accomplish this was by identifying their true element.

By applying my "Bonnie Theory," I was able to identify their true element and guide them to a different exercise that was right for their element type. At the same time, it created a more ambient atmosphere for our team. It was a win-win.

My team was finally performing at their best. They were happy because they started giving their competitors a run for their money and winning races. One time we beat a top team, and their coach was so flabbergasted he reprimanded them for losing to us. We went on to defeat another top team. After the race, that coach jokingly asked me if the course that we created was measured accurately because it appeared to be short.

At the close of the second season, the athletic director looked at the academic grade averages of all the teams. Our team placed the highest with the best grade point average. The "Bad News Bears" were finally proud of what they were doing.

At the end of the season, they gave me a scrapbook filled with memorabilia that captured magical moments in our training and races. It was titled, "The Bad News Bears."

SUCCESS STORIES

Let me share two inspirational stories of how my theory helped my former athletes. One found the right exercise, and the other found he could do more than one type of exercise and do it well.

-GRACE THE RUNNER-

Grace, one my first scholarship athletes, was referred to me by her high school coach. He and I chatted a few times about the many good qualities she possessed. The coach believed that she would make a good candidate as a team player coupled with impressive race times.

I scheduled a meeting with Grace to offer her a scholarship, and we were off to a good start, or so I thought.

When I watched Grace run, she looked like she was pushing a donkey up a hill. Grace was much slower than I imagined she would be. There was no spring in her step and she always wore a painful smile on her face. On top of that, she was always late to practices. Her grades were suffering, she wasn't winning races, and she was getting minor injuries. OMG!

When I had the team swimming and running in the

water, she was the most outstanding swimmer out of the group. Water seemed to be a natural medium for her. She looked happier swimming than running. That painful smile was replaced with a happy one.

I decided to have a conference with her. Grace was so sensitive; she was almost in tears at the thought of being reprimanded for her poor performances. Her sensitive personality was my first clue to what I thought her true element was.

We chatted about her problems with running, and what was going on in her life. She reluctantly shared her concern about continuing to run.

I asked her how it was that she performed so well in high school and not now? The explanation was that running in high school was easier for her. Grace went on to explain that her mother was a renowned runner in college and her goal was to follow in mom's footsteps. Now that Grace was running at a more advanced level, she couldn't cut the mustard.

At this point, I needed to help her find the right exercise, so I asked if she was willing to take-a-peek at my "Bonnie Theory."

Grace read the information,

and I asked which element she felt most cozy with. Tears streamed down her face as she identified with the Water Element.

Running isn't an exercise that water elements are inclined to do. Grace confessed that she had been swimming with a couple of gals on the swim team, and that she felt more connected to swimming than running.

Grace said she was thinking about giving up her running scholarship but felt she would be letting her mom, me, and the team down. Now that Grace found her true element, she was confident that this decision would be the right one.

> ***"You can only become truly accomplished at something you love." Maya Angelou*** [22]

We spoke to the women's head swim coach, and he was open to the idea of her joining the women's swim team. He had her try out to see if she had qualifying times to race. Bingo! This runner transformed into a mermaid, and to her delight, they trained in the

---

[22] https://www.goodreads.com/quotes/4749-you-can-only-become-truly-accomplished-at-something-you-love

afternoon, which is the time most Water Elements prefer.

Grace became injury free and was one of the top finishers in her races. A sweet smile replaced her painful smile. Her healthy ego returned as she began to live in the present moment. Grace was swimming upstream, not downstream. Her body, mind, and spirit were finally one. The problems that plagued her when running were no longer troubling her. She was scot-free.

Once in an interview, she told the media that I not only trained my runners, but that I tuned into their mental aspect as well. Grace also said I had the ability to key into their problems, for which she was grateful.

-DENNIS THE ROWER-

Here's another story of an athlete that benefited by using my "Bonnie Theory".

Dennis was referred to me by his rowing coach who, at one time, was an Olympian, and a friend of mine. The buzz around the campus was that he was an incredible coach. This coach, and I had conversed in the past about the evolution of my new theory. I shared with him the good fortune my athletes were experiencing by using it.   My friend was so impressed, that he wanted me to meet with one of his student athletes, Dennis, and show him my concept. The coach felt that Dennis was not performing up to his ability and wanted him to join my cross-country team to strengthen his performance in rowing.   Dennis was opposed to the idea and didn't understand how it could help.

I scheduled a meeting with Dennis, and he was not a happy camper. He was stubborn, pissed off, indecisive, and impatient. On top of that, he wouldn't make eye contact with me.

This stubborn yet sensible

young man said he didn't want to give up rowing, and I explained that he wouldn't have to. There would be no conflict because the two sports were not played in the same season. He was relieved to hear that.

My instinct was that Dennis would be a perfect fit with the Earth Element as he would be able to do both ground and water exercises. I shared my theory with him and asked if he would look through my booklet to see which of the four elements, he identified with.

Dennis reluctantly admitted that he resonated most with the

descriptive characteristics of the Earth Element. Our eyes made contact for the very first time since we met. I was blown away by this moment. My instinct was confirmed. I was delighted because once an Earth Element commit to something you can rely on them to complete it. Realizing he could do both water and ground exercises, made him more at ease and receptive to doing cross-country.

As Dennis began running with the team, he took to the sport quickly and was a joy to watch. His emotional nature settled down and became more trusting of me. Finding his true element was an important revelation. To his amazement he really enjoyed running as much as he liked rowing.

Dennis was getting stronger; mentally, emotionally, and physically. I knew that when rowing season started, he was going to have a good one. He came to the realization that he needed to be more open to changes in the future.

As time progressed, he became a role model for the other team members. His discipline in training showed in his running times. Dennis followed the rules, his teammates admired him, and he worked well with the female team captain. I asked him if he would like to be the men's team captain for the next season, and he was honored to accept the role. Happy and content, I was on my way to building quality cross-country teams. A little bit of heaven…

When looking back, I could see his image surge up a steep hill leading a pack of runners with ease yelling to him, "Go Dennis!" To watch him run was like experiencing poetry in motion. It gave me goose bumps.

"The highest level of performance comes to people who are centered, intuitive, and reflective –who know how to see a problem as an opportunity." **Deepak Chopra**[23]

---

[23] brainyquote.com/quotes/deepak_chopra_599953

He was a hard worker, organized, stable as a table, and very loyal. After one of our meets, I was driving the bus home and kept hearing requests to stop for a restroom break. Suddenly I heard Dennis yell out, "If you can't hold your liquor, you shouldn't be drinking." This was his way of informing me there was liquor on board.

Dennis proved his loyalty to me and to his team as the situation was handled with kid gloves. He alerted me to the problem without giving any names. I thought it was wise of him.

I immediately pulled over and asked who was drinking. One of them stated they were only drinking apple juice.   Oh, boy. The bad news bears once again reared their ugly heads, but the incident never happened again. When Dennis was interviewed by the media, they quoted him as saying, "This year is so much different.   Everyone is motivated and dedicated to giving 100% every time they run. Coach Frankel really believes and trusts her runners. She's definitely one of the finest coaches we have at the school".

When rowing was back in season, I sat with his coach to watch one of Dennis' races. The coach was quick to notice the positive impact that running had on his performance as a rower. Running had made Dennis stronger, coupled with more endurance. In the eyes of his coach, he was measuring up to his full potential.

He continued to do both sports. Dennis liked the fact that under his element, he could do ground or water related exercises. It wouldn't have surprised me, if he went on to doing a triathlon. Dennis was able to learn a valuable lesson. He learned not to let his fear of change prevent him from launching new opportunities that would better his circumstances in certain situations in life.

"To improve is to change;
to be perfect is to change often."
Winston Churchill[24]

---

[24] https://www.goodreads.com/quotes/44835-to-improv

WOMEN'S SWIM TEAM

When the cross-country teams ended its season, I was approached by the athletic director to take over the helm for another problem team. This was the good news. He was in a quandary because the women's head swim coach quit just as their season was about to begin. The swim team was left in the lurch with no one to coach them. That was the bad news.

The athletic director had been very impressed with the success the cross-country teams had shown in such a short period of time. He felt that I could be an inspiration for the swim team because of my enthusiasm and leadership. The director complimented me by saying he felt my charismatic and warm personality would fire them up, so they could finish their season.

Once more I stepped up to the plate and accepted the challenge. At least they had a team, whereas the cross-country teams had next to none. That was the good news.

The assistant coach was still on board, but the athletes didn't like her. Why would they? The swim team didn't like themselves. They were angry and hurt because their coach walked out on them.

A sense of abandonment plagued their state of mind making them feel nobody cared about them. The swim team was emotionally, mentally, and physically in turmoil.

They were being surly and cynical with me when I took over their coaching. They wouldn't listen to me and were always goofing off during what should have been practice time. What to do? What to do? Aside from abandonment issues, they just quit on themselves and weren't motivated to do anything except, maybe show up, goof off and moan.

The quick fix was to get them to do swim workouts, walk or run once a week, and work as a team. Most of the swimmers had been swimming since they were wee ones and had enough experience to train on their own. They just chose not to.

Being defiant was at the top of their list. Cooperation was like pulling teeth. They complained about any training suggestion I made. Playing mind games with me was what seemed to give them the most pleasure.

One time, when driving the bus on our way to a race, I asked them which freeway exit to take? They just toyed with me by giving me the silent treatment.

I finally yelled at them, "That's it! If you can't tell me which exit to turn off, I'm going to park the bus in the middle of the freeway until I get a response." As I started to do so, I heard a very meek voice from the back, "You get off at the next exit."

After this incident, I figured it was time to take control and share my secret with them. There were many ways I could have worked with the swim team on a one on one basis, but I needed a quick remedy to get them ready for racing. So, the next best solution was to use a group effort approach to the "Bonnie Theory".

Since swimmers are typically water elements, I appealed to two of their positive personality traits. They are creative and sentimental, treasuring their past experiences. I challenged them to come up with favorite workouts they liked doing with their previous coaches, and we would use those to train with.

The lack of exercise would only bring out their negative personality and emotional traits, whereas exercising would bring their positive traits into harmonious alignment.   No matter what happens, I promised not to abandon them. My commitment was to help them be the best they could be as a group. They just needed to finish the season and swim their hearts out to stay fit, physically and psychologically. Let the games begin!

By the time swim season ended, they were healthier, fit, happy, and more bonded as a team. They were able to complete the swim season, which was a big accomplishment for them, and for me as well. They even bonded with the assistant coach. The athletic director was ecstatic, and a new swim coach was hired. When the new coach asked what I did to keep them so fit, I simply told him to run or walk them once a week.

MY PERSONAL CHALLENGE

Coaching young athletes like these helped validate my theory. I was no longer the only one to benefit from finding the right exercise. The positive changes that took place in all areas of their lives warmed my soul.

Once I had accomplished setting a concrete theory in motion, I wanted to take on my reoccurring goal to qualify for the Olympic Trials and inspire others to follow my lead.

"The most important thing is to try and inspire people so that they can be great in whatever they do," Kobe Bryant[25]

My continued quest to go for the gold became a daring priority. I wanted to be a role model to inspire others to pursue dreams they only dared to dream. I wanted to show them that it was the process not necessarily the goal itself that was important. The process would take one to a better place in life or open doors that they never thought could be opened even if you didn't accomplish the goal.

---

[25] https://www.brainyquote.com/quotes/kobe_bryant_574704

I had been thinking about leaving the coaching job at Loyola Marymount, so I could finally devote quality time to train for the Olympic Trials. Loyola and I were not seeing eye to eye about discipling the disruptive members of my team. The final straw was when they pushed the pedal to the metal. Two of the female big wigs from the athletic department brought me into a small office and told me I needed to wear a bra.

That was it! I told them it was more important to maintain team rules than it was for me to wear a bra. So, no rules, no bra! I got fired.

When I told a friend of mine, who was a prominent coach in our conference, that I was leaving he said, "Loyola is really going to miss you. You have a real gift. Your coaching style is unique, and you get great results by connecting with your athletes individually, and as a team. You raised the bar in coaching and made the other schools wake up and take notice."

Other schools offered me head coaching jobs in running (cross-country and track and field) but I decided to devote my time to qualify for the Olympic Trials. It was time for my personal challenge.

AN OLYMPIC GOAL

While training for my goal, I had to find a way to pay the bills. The thought crossed my mind, why not be a personal trainer? It would be easier to train others one-on-one and set my own hours.

I made sure my "Bonnie Theory" booklet was up to date. My clients could look it over, and choose which element they most identified with. Then I could evaluate them to see if we were on the same page. If we disagreed, we would try both elements to see which fit best.

One of my private clients was a

stay-at-home mom named Rika. She was also a serious writer trying to spread her wings. Rika battled a lifelong weight problem. Doom and gloom seemed to be her mantra. She couldn't lose weight no matter how hard she tried.

When we met, she was doing circuit training at a local gym because her husband had recommended this type of exercise. I asked her if it was working. "No progress," was her reply. To up the ante, her husband offered to give her a thousand dollars for a new wardrobe if she lost her designated ten pounds.

This aroused my curiosity. He

felt that she would do best in accomplishing this task if she did the exercise that worked for him; which was circuit training. Many people tend to do exercises that have worked for others with hopes it will do the same for them. It's the old story…monkey see, monkey do, works for me, works for you.

Rika was getting frustrated not meeting her goal, and her old inner ego kept whispering, "Why bother? I feel I'm wasting my time and I'm not even enjoying it." Her ego was living in the past because she could never accomplish this feat, and the future didn't look promising. She was not dealing with the now.

Always looking for the right way to lose weight with foods, she'd go on line, buy different books, and try different diets. Rika was so focused on using the latest fads to lose weight that it never occurred to her that she simply had not found the right exercise.

The right exercise would have had her negative ego tweet a different message in her head allowing her to associate with exercise in a positive way. She would have been happy, and the pounds would have automatically peeled off. Since circuit training is indicative of an earth element, the question was, "Was she truly an earth element?"

Rika was going to be in for a major revelation. I was going to help her find the exercise that fit her true element and would put a positive spin on her life.

"Love what you do and do what you love. Don't listen to anyone else who tells you not to do it. You do what you want, what you love. Imagination should be the center of your life." Ray Bradbury[26]

---

[26] https://www.goodreads.com/quotes/547018-love-what-you-do-and-do-what-you-love-don-t

I told her about my theory of the elements and once more, pulled out my handy booklet. As Rika looked at the four elements with a surprised look, she said, "Woops! I guess circuit training is my husband's thing, not mine."

She quickly identified with the Air Element. Rika tried a few of the exercises under this element and found to her delight that walking was a great fit for her. The longer the walk, the better she felt. It was a life-style habit she would look forward to doing. She treated herself to the latest state of the art smart watch to even make her walk more enjoyable and functionable.

Most people complain about not having enough time to exercise, but she was bright and found a way to combine her exercise, errands, her writing, and many other tasks at the same time. Walking gave her the freedom to think about the book she was working on in hopes of it becoming a best seller.

After losing ten pounds and winning her bet, she and her husband had a good laugh. They ended up using the money for a household emergency instead of a new wardrobe.

"Walking is the best possible exercise. Habituate

yourself to walk very far."
Thomas Jefferson.[27]

Rika was able to release much of her emotional turmoil. When interacting with her children and husband, she was more tolerant of their needs. The positive traits of her personality and emotions became more dominant as she continued to walk.

When doing the right exercise, her personality traits and her emotional reactions were supporting her life style in an enlightened way. She looked more beautiful as if that could be

---

[27] http://www.quotationspage.com/quote/3020.html

possible. Her children were happier, and her husband admired her achievement. What was even more phenomenal, her ego was not locked in the negative murmurs from the past. It was able to tweet a pleasant present and the future felt promising.

In addition to helping Rika, I began coaching her kids, Rob and Isabella. One was eight and the other was ten. These youngsters were able to find the right exercise and reap the benefits at an early stage in their life. Rika wanted her kids to be ahead of the game. Satisfaction filled my soul. Pairing people with their personal element, coupled with the right exercise, works well for any age. Getting a jump start at a young age begins the alignment of exercise with the fitness of your mind and body.

While continuing to personal train others with my newly launched theory, I was also training very hard to reach my own goal. In the process of training to qualify for the 2000 Olympic Trials, my racing times were inconsistent, and I started to develop a slight limp. Even though I was winning races, I was not meeting the qualifying times.

While continuing to train, fate was not on my side. I was hit by a car in an underground parking garage. The doctor took x-rays, and I was diagnosed with Sickle Cell Anemia disease (also known as "Bo Jackson's Disease"). The doctors couldn't believe I was running races and training on a hip that was bone on bone.

I ended up having a hip replacement in the year of 2000 and never thought I would walk let alone run again. Deciding to take charge of my own physical rehabilitation, I was able to get back to training to everyone's amazement, including my own.

*"**Success is walking from failure to failure with no loss of enthusiasm.**" **Winston Churchill**[28]*

To help with my lengthy recovery in the year of 2001, I decided to move to a friend's home in Palm Springs. I continued to train, and my strength and speed returned. It was 2004, and the Olympic Trials were ready for me to try qualifying one more time.

Once again, fortune was against me. My qualifying times were still not fast enough. I felt like Rocky Balboa from the movie Rocky. Disappointment set in by not accomplishing my dream. I felt

---

[28] https://www.democraticunderground.com/12528564

unsuccessful at being a role model to inspire others to follow their dreams. However, I never gave up on the exercise meant for me…running.

"Success is not final; failure is not fatal: it is the courage to continue that counts." Winston Churchill[29]

Whether or not I met my goal, I knew down deep that I would still find a way to inspire people through my new-found theory. My

---

[29]https://www.brainyquote.com/quotes/winston_churchill _124653

belief was that continuous training

would always keep me fit in all areas of my life.

"I do it as a therapy. I do it as something to keep me alive. We need a little discipline. Exercise is my discipline." Jack LaLanne[30]

---

[30] https://www.brainyquote.com/quotes/jack_lalanne_258810

PSYCOLOGICAL MAKEUP: How It Relates to Exercise

"We don't see things as they are, we see them as we are." *Anais Nin* [31]

What is it about our psychological make up that plays an important role in finding the right exercise? Do you ever wonder why your significant other loves to bike and you would rather swim?

Human behavior underlies

---

[31]https://www.goodreads.com/quotes/5030-we-don-t-see-things-as-they-are-we-see-them

almost everything we do, from exercise to politics. This means that our own underlying psychological structure shapes how and why we choose the exercises we do.

This consistent, psychological makeup plays a huge part in defining what exercises work best with an individual. It helps you choose an exercise that you will love and stick with.

Your psychological makeup is defined by two components: 1) your personality traits, such as being daring, imaginative or practical; and 2) your emotional characteristics, such as joy, frustration or anger.

"Personality and emotions go hand in hand and it's often hard to separate the two. Personality is to emotion as climate is to weather."[32]

Climate is a steady factor and weather changes all the time. One sees your personality but observes different emotions at any given moment.

F. Scott Fitzgerald once remarked, "Personality is a

---

[32]https://personality-project.org/revelle/publications/ets.2003.pdf

series of successful gestures."[33]

Personality is made up of the characteristic patterns of thoughts and behaviors that make a person unique.   People identify you by your personality. For example; being stubborn, outspoken or gentle; he's adventurous, she's creative, he is a pioneer, she's a hard worker.

Personality has an influence on the type of exercise you choose, and in turn exercise affects your personality. Let's use myself as an example: I can be fidgety and

---

[33]https://blog.ginsudo.com/2007/11/14/personality-is-an-unbroken-series-of-successful-gestures/

somewhat impatient due to my element's personality traits, but when I run, it releases my negativity and shifts it into a more positive gear. It lifts my spirits, clears my head and helps me deal with life's problems in a more harmonious way. I call it an active form of meditation.

When you find the right element that best defines you, the exercise you choose will align with the positive part of your personality. It helps develop the mind and body connection as well as keeping you physically fit.

So, does this mean that the physical exercises you are drawn to are a result of your personality? Or do your personality traits develop because of those physical exercises? I think it's both.

Now let us consider the emotional side of your psychological makeup. Keep in mind, your personality and emotional traits closely interact in the way they affect your psyche. Sometimes it's hard to tell the difference between the two.

People identify you by your personality, but your emotions are instinctive reactions. Emotions have a wide range depending on your surroundings and how you relate to others.

There are two 19th century psychologists, American William James and the Danish physician Dr. Carl Lange, that independently developed what is now known as the "James-Lang Theory".[34]   It explains that emotions are the result of an external stimulus, producing a physiological response.

In 2014, Dr. Rachael Jack, from the Neuroscience & Psychology University in Glasgow, also did a study. It states that in fact, there are only four fundamental emotions; fear, happy,

---

[34]http://www.everything.explained.today/James–Lange theory/

sad, and anger."[35]

Emotions organize our thinking and response to different types of challenges. So, let's look at these four emotions and how they affect us because exercise will play an important role with them.

FEAR is a powerful emotion that was critical in keeping our primitive ancestors alive and continues to be vital to our very existence. It warns us of eminent or threatening danger that might be harmful.

There are two responses to fear, biochemical, and emotional.

---

[35]https://www.spring.org.uk/2014/02/how-many-basic-emotions-are-there-fewer-than-was-previously-thought.php

Physically, we break out in a sweat, our heart rate goes up and, our adrenaline starts pumping. We then go into a "fight or flight" response. It is an involuntary response that we rely on to keep us safe.

"The only thing we have to fear is fear itself." Franklin D. Roosevelt[36]

The emotional response to fear is different for everyone. It is either positive or negative depending on the situation. The infamous painting of Edvard

---

[36] http://historymatters.gmu.edu/d/5057

Munch, "The Scream," captures the very essence of this emotion. It expresses how fear can be paralyzing, making us unable to deal with threatening situations. Fear can also be fun, like watching a scary movie, and there are those adrenaline junkies that thrive on fear to make them feel exhilarated, like sky diving.

"Do one thing every day that scares you." Eleanor Roosevelt[37]

HAPPINESS is a delicious

---

[37]https://www.goodreads.com/quotes/25106-do-one-thing-every-day-that-scares-you

emotion which can keep you content and healthy. People who are happy are more apt to exercise and stick with it. Learning new things come easily when you're happy. It also keeps you in a positive frame of mind.

When you find yourself feeling sad, angry or fearful, try to replace it with some activity that pleases you such as watching a funny movie or seeing something beautiful or engaging in an exercise you love to perform. This will help you escape those negative emotions.

"*Can feeling too good ever*

be bad? "June Gruber[38]

Too much happiness can make you less creative and less safe." June Gruber[39]

The desire for achieving a prolonged nirvana, can lead to risky behaviors such as excessive alcohol consumption, binge-eating, and drug abuse.

"Happiness may be best

---

[38]
https://www.dallasnews.com/opinion/commentary/2012/06/01/june-gruber-the-dark-side-of-happiness

[39]https://webwriterspotlight.com/happiness-can-make-you-less-creative-competitive

when experienced in moderation - not too little, but also not too much." **June Gruber**[40]

SADNESS is an uncomfortable emotion. It is thought of as a negative emotion but does serve an important purpose. You need to accept sadness as a part of your emotional makeup. It can be a mild signal telling you that something challenging in your life needs to be addressed.

---

[40]

https://greatergood.berkeley.edu/article/item/four_ways_happiness_can_hurt_you

Happy people are sometimes less motivated to push forward, whereas someone experiencing sadness will be **more** motivated to change their unpleasant situation.

When people are sad, they tend to be more sensitive to what surrounds them and are more creative than when they are happy. This can be seen in many artists' works.

Often when we watch sad movies or listen to sad music it makes us cry. This helps us to release negative feelings. Being sad can improve our memory, enable us to be less judgmental, and less bias. When all is said and done, sadness helps us appreciate the times we are happy.

"The word 'happy' would lose its meaning if it were not balanced by sadness." Carl Jung.[41]

ANGER is a vital secondary emotion. It is a response to other emotions felt first that triggers anger. An angry response is often used to protect or cover up vulnerable feelings.

Since anger is part of our human experience, we feel it in different ways and at different levels. We get angry due to a combination of factors: trigger

---

[41]https://quotation.io/page/quote/word-happy-lose-meaning-balanced-sadness

events, individual characteristics, and how we appraise any given situation.

"Feelings can't be ignored no matter how unjust or ungrateful they seem." Anne Frank.[42]

A trigger event could be such as being insulted. We first feel defensive, and then we get angry. If a person has the characteristic of being possessive, they are likely to become angry if they feel threatened or if something vital will be taken from them. We can also

---

[42]https://themindsjournal.com/but-feelings-cant-be-ignored/

get angry when we appraise a situation and feel it is unjust or unfair.

"What I've learned about being angry with people is that it generally hurts you more than it hurts them." Oprah Winfrey[43]

Some things that trigger anger are injustice, criticism, frustration, or simply not getting our way. Anger can range from mild irritation to seething rage. That's why it's important to be able to control our anger. So, is anger good or bad? The answer is in the

---

[43]https://www.azquotes.com/quote/544082

following quote.

"Anger is good, and anger can also be bad. Anger is a God-given emotional feeling or energy designed for good, but the way we use and express our anger-produced energy can often be dysfunctional." Dr. Karl Benzio[44]

In general, exercising gives you the tools to deal with your emotions. It helps alleviate emotions that are worrisome, such as, anger, sadness or fear, and

---

[44] lighthousenetwork.org/2017/07/anger-good-bad/

encourages happiness because of the endorphins it releases.

"There are times when I feel lazy and just want to stay in bed all day, but I know that working out is the best way to get those endorphins going which make me feel better emotionally and physically" **Heather Locklear.**[45]

Exercise puts you in a right frame of mind by boosting your resilience to a negative situation before it can occur. It is nature's way to manage emotion. The pharmaceutical industry has tried to

---

[45] https://www.allgreatquotes.com/quote-176916/

manufacture a pill like this for decades.

"Emotion arises at the place where mind and body meet. It is the body's reaction to your mind." Eckhardt Tolle[46]

If you are sad, you might cry. If you are angry, you might hit something. Your body responds to the way you think and feel. When you're stressed, your body might raise your blood pressure to let you know something is wrong. This is a form of a mind and body connection.

---

[46] https://www.allgreatquotes.com/quote-176916/

Your mind can send the body messages like, "I don't like this exercise…" It's too hard… no fun", and so on. As a result, your body gives in and stops doing it.

If the mind has influence over the body, what is it that controls the mind? It's our ego. It sets up our emotions with good or bad results. So, allow me to introduce you to another way of looking at this part of our inner self.

"The term ego means different things to different people, but when I use it, it means a false self that is created by unconscious identification

with the mind. To the ego, the present hardly exists. Only past and future are considered important." Eckhardt Tolle.[47]

Most people think of ego when we see a person bragging about themselves. We think, "What a big ego that person has." Well, there's more to ego than just being a braggart.

The ego is an inner voice that speaks to your mind all the time. It can be negative or positive. An unhealthy ego keeps you thinking about the past or future and does

---

[47]https://www.facebook.com/AustraliansCounselof13Grandm others/posts/1615381628493725

not keep you in the present. It can have you relive all the negative experiences you have had and make the future seem unattainable.

An unhealthy ego is also the biggest reason people don't exercise. If you've had a negative experience with exercise in the past, your ego keeps whispering to your mind, questioning, "Why bother? It hasn't worked for me in the past, why would it work for me now?" With this kind of negative thinking, it's amazing a person would try to exercise at all let alone try something new.

The opposite is also true. When the mind responds to an exercise you like, your emotions are more positive, satisfied, and pleased. Your body starts looking forward to being physically active and the fitness begins as you repeat the process.

"It is exercise alone that supports the spirits and keeps the mind in vigor.… our minds are rendered buoyant by exercise." Marcus Tullius Cicero.[48]

Being physically active enhances and re-enforces a positive

---

[48]https://www.azquotes.com/author/2894-Marcus_Tullius_Cicero/tag/exercise

psychological makeup. It interrupts the old negative patterns that whisper to your subconscious mind. So, when you find the right element, it will help you choose an exercise that is cooked just right for your palate. The voice of the ego will become more positive and will replace negative murmurs. That's why finding the right exercise is so important.

"True enjoyment comes from activity of the mind and exercise of the body. The two are ever united." **Wilhelm von**

Humboldt [49]

---

[49]

https://www.brainyquote.com/quotes/wilhelm_von_humboldt_
141400

NOT JUST DIET ALONE

What will benefit you more? The right exercise or just diet alone? Diet by itself won't cut it. Fitness, not weight is the important factor in health. Just being thin does not equal fitness.

"If you don't exercise you won't attain fitness." Bonnie Frankel

People gain weight when they over eat and don't exercise. The body is like a car. It needs to be used on a regular basis to keep it in good working condition. You wouldn't overfill the gas tank to keep your car running, so why would you want to overfeed your body? If you don't drive your car and let it sit for a while, the engine won't start. If you don't exercise, your body machine may not function.

*"**A muscle is like a car. If you want it to run well early in the morning, you have to warm it up." Florence Griffith-Joiner.**[50]*

---

[50] www.searchquotes.com/quotation/A_muscle_is_like_a_car._If_you_want_it_to_run_well_early_in_the_morning%2C_you_have_to_warm_it_up./116247/

You do need to watch what you eat, but you must also move your body to burn unwanted calories. Just as with exercise, there is no one-fits-all diet. Diets are typically designed for the masses whether it's in the form of food types, protein drinks or diet pills.

I saw this on a T-shirt. It struck my funny bone.

"Did you know DIET stands for: Did I eat that?" [51]

Your goal should be fitness, not just hitting a goal weight. Exercising creates a different spin

---

[51] https://www.gearbubble.com/did-you-know-diet-tshirt

on eating. Being active will help you make better choices with your diet and you won't crave junk food.

"Pay attention to your body. The point is everybody is different. You have to figure out what works for you." *Andrew Weil[52]*

Let's check out why people gain weight in the first place. It's simple. If you consume more than you need to run your body, it will store extra calories as fat. These fat deposits function as a reserve in the event we miss a meal or two.

[52]https://www.brainyquote.com/quotes/andrew_weil_202295

However, if someone consistently over eats, the body will store too many calories which will lead to becoming overweight. Exercise is the key to stopping this fat storage.

"*Every time I lose weight, I find it in the refrigerator.*" *Minion life quotes.*[53]

Even though being an advocate for Weight Watchers, Jennifer Hudson still exercised five days a week to lose eighty pounds.

The prime cause of weight gain is a result of behavior. If your

---

[53]http://www.lovethispic.com/image/336598/every-time-i-lose-some-weight,-i-find-it-again-in-the-refrigerator

emotions are in a negative place, you'll go to food for emotional gratification. Food will become the focus of your attention and your body and mind will become addicted to eating. You'll start using food to satisfy what's lacking in your life, and the cravings will begin.

Here's another funny T-shirt quote.

"If stress burned calories, I'd be a super model." Minion life quotes.[54]

Your daily life has many

---

[54] https://www.cafepress.com/ifstressburnedcalories

emotional triggers. Eating is a way to suppress or soothe negative emotions. It's even possible for those negative emotions to be expressed by physical illnesses, and in psychological disorders.

"Those who do not find time for exercise will have to find time for illness." Earl of Derby[55]

My dad always said, "You can take a trip to get away from your problems but those same problems are still waiting for you when you return." Exercise helps relieve the

---

[55]https://www.coursehero.com/file/11254776/Chapter-13-Exercise/

stress of the problems without having to escape them with the expense of a trip.

So, it is with weight gain. You can diet and lose, but eventually it comes back. With diets, you may drop pounds but when you plateau, you'll become disinterested. As a result, you dump the diet and drop back into old habits.

"Dear stomach, you're bored not hungry. So, shut up." Minion life quotes[56]

Food obsession makes you lose

---

[56]www.lovethispic.com/image/234739/dear-stomach,-you%27re-bored,-not-hungry.-so-shut-up

your freedom of choice. When you eat to feed your emotions, the biochemistry of the brain starts calling the shots.

John J. Ratey, explained in his book, "Spark: The Revolutionary New Science of Exercise and the Brain," that moving our muscles produces proteins that travel through the blood stream and into the brain where they play pivotal roles in the mechanisms of our highest thought processes.

"We must go beyond the constant clamor of ego, beyond the tools of logic and reason, to the still, calm place within us; the realm of the soul." Deepak

Chopra[57]

Without exercise the brain, or whispering ego, will keep telling you things like, "Just one more bite won't hurt". "I'm not full yet". "I'm fat anyway, so why not eat?" Sound familiar?

Then, after you eat those extra calories, you'll chastise yourself because you can't control your eating habits. Well, they are just that, habits. It's like chasing your own tail. Dieting alone gives you a false goal. You can lose a couple of

---

[57] https://www.brainyquote.com/quotes/deepak_chopra_599956

pounds, but diet doesn't cancel out the emotional urge to eat.

"Don't forget you are what you eat. I need to eat a skinny person," Anonymous[58]

The best way to interrupt the eating syndrome is to replace it with an alternative activity. Choose something that you'd look forward to doing. When connecting with an exercise that coincides with your true element, it disrupts the urge to eat. Taking care of your body and mind is important because they are

---

[58]quotespictures.com/dont-forget-you-are-what-you-eat-i-need-to-eat-skinny-person-clever-quotes/

the only ones you have.

You must be physically active and by doing the right exercise keeps your mind in the right place as well as keeping your body fit, not fat.

Whether you're over or under weight, most of us need physical activity to release our feelings. Exercising releases endorphins that calm our minds. Today's society carries way too much stress and frustration. When you do the right exercise that fits your psychological makeup, it allows emotional debris to discharge from your brain, so you can confront everyday challenges in a better way. If we take care of ourselves in the right way, we will live well beyond our ancestors' expectations.

Diets address portion control and the type of food you eat, but it doesn't erase the cravings for carbs, fats and sugars. Exercise speeds up your metabolism and stops these cravings. A faster metabolism also helps you burn the excess fat and calories. Thus, you'll eat healthier and drink more fluids.

And finally, those of you who are underweight need to exercise because being skinny is not being fit either. When you exercise you won't have the emotional feeling that you're putting on weight.

Physical activity will be burning calories and create an appetite by stimulating the palate. It will rid you of those emotions that have stopped you from eating in the past.

"Human bodies are designed for regular physical activity. The sedentary nature of much of modern life probably plays a significant role in the epidemic incidence of depression today. Many studies show that depressed patients who stick to a regimen of aerobic exercise improve as much as those treated with medication."

Andrew Weil [59]

So, in reference to diets, you are actually better off exercising to let the pounds fall off naturally, and your choices of foods and liquids will be healthier. Choosing the right exercise will help you achieve the goal of fitness and health.

Now it's time to help you identify which element you are…Fire, Air, Earth or Water. Take the following quiz to find out.

---

[59] https://www.inspiringquotes.us/quotes/duh0_crgT564y

FINDING YOUR ELMENT

QUIZ

PERSONALITY TRAITS

In each group, circle one word that best describes your personality

Do you consider yourself as…?

    a) Unpredictable

    b) Objective

    c) Sensible

    d) Compassionate

When you're meeting people for the first time are you…?

    a) Outspoken

    b) A chatterbox

    c) Cordial

    d) A quiet listener

Do others see you as…?

a) A leader

b) An organizer

c) Stable

d) Friendly

Is your personality…?

a) Charismatic

b) Clever

c) Decisive

d) Creative

How do you deal with problems?

a) Impulsively

b) Analyze it

c) Logically

d) Go with the flow

Does the opposite sex find you…?

a) Energetic

b) Charming

c) Loyal

d) Nurturing

EMOTIONAL TRAITS

In each group, Circle one reaction you might have that best describes your motions.

If you won the lottery would you...?

a) Run around in circles

b) Share it with others

c) Start planning how to invest your money

d) Cry uncontrollably with joy

If your best friend blocked you from Facebook, would you…?

 a) Feel it was probably your fault

 b) Remove them

 c) Find out why

 d) Feel devastated

When your boss is treating you unfairly would you…?

 a) Give the boss a piece of your mind

 b) Schedule a meeting

 c) Try to work harder

 d) Keep quiet and steam inside

If an argument broke out would you…?

a) Be ready to punch anyone that threatened you

b) Step aside and analyze the situation

c) Try to talk sense into the offenders

d) Try to pacify the situation

TYPES OF EXERCISES YOU MIGHT LIKE

In each group, Circle one exercise or sport you might like to do

Group 1

a) Sprinting

b) Cross Country

c) Triathlons

d) Swim

Group 2

a) Fast Walking

b) Jogging

c) Martial Arts

d) Creative Dance

Group 3

a) Zumba

b) Gymnastics

c) Rock Climbing

d) Yoga

Group 4

a) Racquet ball

b) Tennis Singles

c) Bodybuilding

d) Surfing

Group 5

a) Basketball

b) Baseball

c) Football

d) Water Polo

Group 6

a) Speed Skating

b) Skateboarding

c) Roller blading

d) Ice Skating

GATHERING RESULTS

Now total up how many A's, B's, C's & D's you have. The letter with the highest number is your true Element.

___   ___   ___   ___

A   B   C   D

Fire   Air   Earth   Water

MEET THE FOUR ELEMENTS

As you progress to the next chapters, you'll read descriptions of each element, their personalities, what triggers their reactions to the four types of emotions, their exercise traits, and the suggested exercises each element prefers to do.

Remember that each of us has sprinklings of all four elements, but only one of them will speak to you loud and clear. Of course, you'll want to focus on your own personal element, but reading about the others will be fun. You'll see how your family and friends connect with a specific element as well.

FIRE ELEMENT

"My mission in life is not to merely survive, but to thrive; and to do so with some passion, some compassion, some humor and some style," Maya Angelou.[60]

Do you look to be in a position of leadership? Do you embrace being the center of attention? Do you inspire others to do the impossible? If you do, then you have found your home with the Fire Element.

---

[60]https://www.passiton.com/inspirational-quotes/7383-my-mission-in-life-is-not-merely-to-survive

The Fire Element is the most extraordinary of all the elements. People who own this element are dynamic and full of piss and vinegar. They say to themselves, "I can and will do the impossible…the unexpected. Just watch me and challenge me."

Being energetic, daring and spontaneous, these highly competitive and enthusiastic beings can't get enough of exploring life.

"I'm a competitive person and I love the challenge of mastering new things."
Sasha Cohen[61]

---

[61] https://topquotesabout.com/quote/im-a-competitive-

They are spirits in motion bouncing from one thing to another. Their explosive bursts of energy persuading them to fearlessly plunge into things they haven't tried. Fire Elements will gladly share their concepts in a spirited and warm manner encouraging others to follow their lead.

***"He who is not courageous enough to take risks will accomplish nothing in life."* Mohammad Ali** [62]

---

person-and-i-love-the-challenge-of-mastering-new-things/

[62]quotefancy.com/quote/758486/Muhammad-Ali-He-who-is-not..

The other elements gather around them anxiously waiting to hear about their most recent escapades. Fire Elements manifest the power of transformation and can change anything from a negative darkness into a positive illumination.

Fire Elements predominantly live in the moment. Every once in a blue moon they can have a blast from their past memory. They are action-oriented and set themselves up with short-term goals on a regular basis. The past rarely has a hold on this speedy element, because once it's behind them, they are on to the next challenge. They thrive on being in the moment not letting past events affect them. At the same time, they can't wait to see what pops up in their future.

"Nothing ever happened in the past, it happened in the now, nothing will even happen in the future; it will happen in the now." Eckhardt Tolle [63]

They are prone to sudden, illuminating flashes of insight with bursts of enthusiastic flare and a passion for life. Fire is infused with

---

[63]https://www.goodreads.com/quotes/396943-nothing-has-happened-in-the-past-it-happened-in-the

a divine spark and it can spread like a wildfire to everyone around them. This leads them to live large and will feel sad by engaging in mundane chores or duties.

Fire was the first element born when the universe was created. They love to literally live off the seat of their pants with a blazing sense of adventure. This element always follows their gut, so when they don't, their sense of pride is devastated feeling they should have known better. It is, without a doubt, the most entertaining of the elements.

Orange and red are the colors associated with the Fire Element.

They are "fired" up and raring to go. One can imagine seeing red and orange flames shooting off their feet when they are sprinting down the track. The Fire Element is indeed, on fire! To inspire is their goal.

With a colorful and uplifting persona, they encourage the other elements to follow their lead to be positive and unafraid to try new exercises.

"Being positive in a negative situation is not naïve. It's leadership." Ralph Marston [64]

---

[64]https://goleansixsigma.com/positive-negative-situation-not-naive-leadership/

You'll find that Fire Elements are very happy-go-lucky but can be impatient and fly off the handle quickly. The good thing is they don't hold grudges and get back to business just as fast. They are quick to respond to whatever you ask and expect that they will insert their foot in their mouth meaning no harm; just being genuinely honest.

A challenge is what lights the Fire Elements' torch, and they can be obsessive compulsive until it is met. They can and will do most distances, but don't look for them to do a long warm up, as they prefer to just cut to the chase and start their workout.

"Oh my God, Zumba is the greatest invention ever for women. I like to exercise, though I do nothing consistently because I get bored and impatient. With Zumba, you're dancing; you're moving your hips... So much fun." Robin Wright[65]

Start, stop, lunge, sprint is all in the vocabulary of the Fire Element. With or without a coach on hand, quick and fast movement is what they thrive on. However, this feisty, courageous element will

____

[65] https://www.brainyquote.com/quotes/robin_wright_695713

attempt other element's exercises just for the challenge and thrill of it. It feeds their soul.

"Life is often compared to a marathon, but I think it is more like being a sprinter; long stretches of hard work punctuated by brief moments in which are given the opportunity to perform our best." Michael Johnson[66]

An example of a true Fire Element would be the compelling

---

[66]

www.searchquotes.com/quotation/Life_is_often_compared_t o_a_marathon%2C_but_I_think_it_is_more_like_being_a_sp rinter%3B_long_stretches_o/98032/

story about my dear cousin. She was always trying one exercise or another from a very young age. If others challenged her to try any form of exercise, she'd jump right on it and stay with it until she aced it. Everyone loved her because of her outgoing personality, highlighted by her spontaneous spirit.

When she was thirty, she decided to take ice skating lessons. She even entered competitions and won several medals. Even though ice skating isn't a Fire Element's sport, she excelled at it.

After nine years of skating, she began falling. It was more than just the slick ice. It also affected her in her every day activities. It was the beginnings of a journey that would be the challenge of her lifetime.

In 1989 She was diagnosed with Epstein Bar Syndrome and in 1994, a diagnosis of multiple sclerosis was confirmed. She ended up with a list of illnesses: MS, heart disease, rotator cuff surgery and had both hips replaced. She felt like a walking, talking petri dish.

The head of rehab at Saint Mary's hospital in Long Beach, California, finally told her she would never walk again. Her response was, "Really? Just watch me." She applied her fired up nature and ten months later, the same head of rehab was blown away when my cousin walked in the center on her own.

My cousin explained to me that MS patients can be very sensitive to heat, so certain types of exercises rose her body temperature too much. In order to keep exercising, she began to do water workouts where the temperature of the water was suitable for her condition. This enabled her to be physically active to this day.

The drive for the love of being in motion, the dare me not to do the impossible, and her enthusiasm helped her to accomplish something that many a person would have given up trying to do. She was fearless and confident about proving herself to be right. After all, the odds were not in her favor.

Today she might not be able to run a race, but she could certainly walk one. That is pure inspiration. I admired her chutzpah and kept her in mind when I came across my own challenges.

"The desire to reach for the stars is ambitious. The desire to reach hearts is wise. "Maya Angelou[67]

---

[67] **https://www.goodreads.com/quotes/60178-the-desire-to-reach-for-the-stars-is-ambitious-the**

PERSONALITY TRAITS FOR FIRE

POSITIVE	NEGATIVE
Natural Leader	Follower
Charismatic	Boring
Spontaneous	Planned
Enthusiastic	Laid-back
Honest	Blunt
Adventurous	Cautious
Inspiring	Uninteresting
Energetic	Spiritless
Competitive	Noncompetitive
Extrovert	Introvert
Warm	Cold

EMOTIOINAL TRIGGERS FOR FIRE

HAPPY: Taking risks

Feeling Free

Being in motion

Inspiring others

ANGER: Being immobile

The word can't

Being lied to

Being bossed

FEAR: Feeling trapped

      Feeling guilty

      Fading into the crowd

      Not making a difference

SAD: Old rules

      Mundane tasks

      Not being unique

      Being stagnant

EXERCISE TRAITS
FOR FIRE

Thrives being in continuous motion

 Doesn't like to warm up

Will exercise any time of the day

Likes to exercise every day

Prefers short distances

Loves intervals

Self-starter

Competes with self

Loves a challenge

Flexible to do any form of exercise

SUGGESTED EXERCISE FOR FIRE

Sprinting

Fast Walking

Aerobics

Spinning

Soccer

Racquetball

Basketball

Speed Skating

Boxing

Tap Dancing

Zumba

AIR ELEMENT

"I would like to be known as an intelligent woman, a courageous woman, a loving woman who teaches by being." Maya Angelou[68]

Think of the Air Element as being associated with the breath of life. It is uncontainable, elusive, invisible, changeable, and swift. If you are an Air Element, you know that everything begins with an idea. Those that belong to this element will share their thoughts with you

---

[68]https://www.goodreads.com/quotes/651266-i-would-like-to-be-known-as-an-intelligent-woman

and the universe, whether you want to hear them or not. It is the element of insight, vision and communication.

Air Elements focus on their gift of gab to communicate their original ideas in a persistent, analytical and carefree way.

"No matter what people tell you, words and ideas change the world." Robin Williams[69]

Although they are anxious to converse, Air Elements don't give a hoot about what you do with the

---

[69]https/mystrengthsandweaknesses.com/no-matter-the-people-tell-you-words-ideas-change-world-robin-williams/

information. They will simply talk until they drop.

The Air Elements have a detached personality expressing their endeavors with a cool objective attitude which is combined with clarity and sharpness.

"I'll let the racquet do the talking." John McEnroe[70]

This is the element of the mind. It has a cleansing power that connects and refreshes the other elements by enlightening them with its intellect. Air is intelligent,

---

[70] https://www.azquotes.com/quote/553323

rational, and academic.

***"I am always ready to learn although I don't always like being taught." Winston Churchill.*[71]**

Since Air Elements are very clever at storytelling, it makes them brilliant speakers and teachers.

Their primary purpose in life is to educate and make the world a better place. They are new age thinkers and would rather instruct an exercise class than take one.

Air Elements are about rebirth

---

[71]www.simplybetterenglish.com/i-always-ready-learn-although-i-not-always-like-taught-winston-churchill/

and renewal and will fight hard for any type of justice. They are, indeed, like the air we breathe shifting their actions in the present to better shape the future. These brain children thrive in the present moment by thinking, trying, or inventing any new concept.

"The quality of your consciousness at this moment is what shapes the future-which can only be experienced as the now." Eckhardt Tolle[72]

If they should choose a form of

---

[72]https://www.inspiringquotes.us/author/8572-eckhart-tolle/about-quality

exercise that enables them to react in the moment, it gives them a break that is needed from their overloaded mind.

"True enjoyment comes from activity of the mind and exercise of the body. The two are ever entwined." Von Humboldt[73]

This dazzling element is the Public Information Officer of the elements. They are wired in such a way that their emotions do not interfere with their vision. Since

---

[73]

https://www.brainyquote.com/quotes/wilhelm_von_humboldt_141400

they are the social creatures of the elements, they enjoy linking up with diverse people to brainstorm new ideas.

Travel is one of their passions and they love to explore new horizons. They are more than capable of lifting us up to see the world with new eyes. Their colors are white and yellow. This expresses purity of the mind and the enlightenment of a new day that brings hope and new vistas.

Air elements enjoy exercises that are either indoors or outdoors. This new age element prefers a long warm up as well as a long stretch before their main work out. Their thinking behind this regime is that it massages the kinks and prevents them from becoming injured. Air Elements also enjoy the pleasure of a lengthy cool down after their workout coupled with a long stretch to go along with it.

They easily take to using the newest techniques, and gadgets available.

"For cardio, I do SoulCycle. I really don't like to run, plus, I have terrible knees and get bored on the elliptical. SoulCycle is basically a dance partly on a bicycle and you burn calories; and it's so fun." Alison

Williams[74]

The Air Element can be creative and graceful like the Water Element however, they avoid exercising in water. Ground exercises are more to their liking. If they choose to walk, they can walk infinitely.

"My grandmother started walking five miles a day when she was sixty. She's ninety-seven now and we don't know where the hell she is." Ellen

---

[74]

https://www.brainyquote.com/quotes/allison_williams_664934

DeGeneres[75]

When I returned to college in my forties, I had a coach who helped me to compete on a collegiate level. She was a marathon Olympian representing her country of Ireland. This grand Irish lassie was a one-of-a-kind distance runner and represents the Air Element to a T.

I inspired her to start an older woman's running group that began training at 5 AM in the morning. She loved instructing and shared her innovative ideas whenever she

---

[75] https://www.brainyquote.com/quotes/ellen_degeneres_131597

was able to.   Teaching was more important to her than her own life history as a famed runner.

"I've learned that people will forget what you said, people will forget what you did, but people will never forget how you made them feel." Maya Angelou[76]

She had the gift of gab, and never missed a beat. This beloved coach once drove me an hour and a half on her motor scooter to compete in a collegiate competition. She talked all the way there, telling me witty stories of her

---

[76] https://www.goodreads.com/quotes/5934-i-ve-learned-that-people-will-forget-what-you-said-people

childhood in Ireland. Although I couldn't hear all of what she was saying because of the wind whipping by us, I still enjoyed her company. My memory of her is very deep with admiration of the visions she shared with me.

PERSONALITY TRAITS FOR AIR

<u>POSITIVE</u>	<u>NEGATIVE</u>
Witty	Bland
Communicator	Quiet
Educator	Student
Analytical	Hasty
Sociable	Withdrawn
Intelligent	Dull
Inquisitive	Uninterested
Persuasive	Ineffective
Visionary	Unrealistic
Ingenious	Uninventive

WHAT TRIGGERS EMOTIONAL REACTIONS FOR AIR

Happy: New technology

Being inventive

Sharing ideas

Intelligent discussions

Anger: Injustice

Being hushed

Being undermined

Being ignored

Fear: Lack of ideas

Not being original

Being too nerdy

Losing their voice

Sadness: To be the last to know

Lack of new ideas

Unable to express self

Not socializing

EXERCISE TRAITS FOR AIR

They're drawn to ground exercises

Indoor or outdoor works for them

Likes to work out early to mid-morning

Likes to coach others

Does not like water workouts

Prefers long warm up before/after workout

Favors middle to long distance

Can chat when they workout

Will try the latest exercise technique

Likes to vary workouts

Prefers long and lengthy stretch before/after workout

SUGGESTED EXERCISE FOR AIR

Middle to long-distance running

Middle to long-distance walking

Middle to long-distance cycling

Baseball

Softball

Tennis

Golf

Gymnastics

Volleyball

Hiking

Spinning Class/SoulCycle

Ballet

EARTH ELEMENT

"All great achievements require time." Maya Angelou"[77]

Are your feet firmly planted on the ground? Do you produce tangible solutions to problems by using logic? Can you be patient, methodical and devoted to producing solid results to attain your goals? If so, welcome home, Earth Element.

This element is concerned with what is real and physical. It is referred to as the "Mother Earth"

---

[77]http://hubbyshome.com/1251/maya-angelou-quote-great-achievements/

of all the elements that represent our very own planet. It encompasses the same life energy that nourishes our Earth and likewise wants to nourish the body with exercise and movement.

The vitality of this element is here to shape, manifest, cultivate and revel in earthly delights. Its gift to the other elements is to give form to their ideas through example. Earth Elements will tend to their own garden and inspire others to make the most of theirs.

Their philosophy is living in the here and-now and believing in what they can see, hear, touch, taste and smell.

"Life gives you plenty of time to do what you want if you stay in the present moment." **Deepak Chopra**[78]

However, they are heavily attached to their past as they consider it to have a direct impact on their future. The "Mother Earth Elements" tend to be very decisive in the way they do things. Their perception of the past brings a strong sense of value to their lives, which can boost their ambition as well as reduce their tendency to feel stuck.

They are as stable as a table and

---

[78]brainyquote.com/quotes/deepak_chopra_453994

are more concerned with their physical well-being than the spiritual. The Earth Element does not waiver in decision making and tends to see everything as black or white. Their laughter can be quite hardy with a contagious tone and are very slow to anger.

This element is gifted with the understanding that a strong will and common sense go a long way to having any undertaking be successful. It provides the building blocks of nature just as builders do for their creations. Once they get going on a project, they are unwaveringly patient at seeing it through to its completion.

Earth Elements have an enormous amount of endurance and strength, which makes them exceptionally qualified when participating in a triathlon, ironman or marathon. This element excels at connecting different forms of exercise into one long workout. Earth Elements will do ground exercises for the most part, but unlike Air Elements, are willing to exercise or to cross-train with water.

"The marathon is an opportunity for redemption. 'Opportunity', because the outcome is uncertain. 'Opportunity' because it is up to

you, and only you, to make it happen." Dean Karnazes.[79]

Dean Karnazes uses a machine called an 'ElliptiGo'. It is an elliptical bicycle combining the best of running, cycling and elliptical trainer to deliver a low-impact, high-performance workout outdoors. It's a standup stride bicycle that you don't pedal, but stride on. This is a good machine for Earth Elements because it allows them to cross-train with less impact on their joints especially when they are training for an ultramarathon, marathon, or an

---

[79] https://www.azquotes.com/quote/1137579

ironman.

These elements are charming, caring, yet smart enough to know you can't live life with your head in the clouds. All choices must be concrete. Earth Element colors are green and brown, which symbolizes their being grounded and focus on continual growth. There are no gray areas in their decisions…they are not risk takers…it is simply one way or the other.

At times they get so focused with getting to the finishing line, they easily lose sight of the journey.

"I am a slow walker, but I

never walk back. Be sure you put your feet in the right place, then stand firm." Abe Lincoln[80]

Although, the Earth Elements tend to be cautious and conservative in their decisions, they are still able to cut loose and appreciate a good time like everyone else.

One can always count on the dependable Earth Elements, as they will never let you down. Their conventional makeup allows them to concentrate on one project at a time and are successful in whatever they put their mind to

---

[80] http://www.quoteswave.com/picture-quotes/71792

accomplishing.

"*I think if you can be a goal-setting person, it makes it easier to stay motivated.*" Dara Torres[81]

I have a contractor friend Curt, that never lacks for work. When he gets a job, he is completely focused on it until it's finished. He gets dead set on meeting the timeline quoted to his customers and rarely goes over it. Curt never takes short cuts and methodically works through any obstacles that come up along the

---

[81] http://cats.quotemaster.org/author/Dara+Torres

way.

Although the amount of physical activity on the job is plentiful, he finds time to do other activities and exercises that keep him fit as well. One time he asked me for some suggestions on which type of exercises were needed to expand his physicality, so I shared my theory on the element types.

Curt found he loves Tae Kwon Do and bodybuilding and is now even thinking of going into some competitions.

PERSONALITY TRAITS FOR EARTH

<u>POSITIVE</u>   <u>NEGATIVE</u>

POSITIVE	NEGATIVE
Reliable	Unstable
Logical	Unreasonable
Decisive	Procrastinates
Stable	Inconsistent
Disciplined	Neglect
Generous	Stingy
Conventional	Informal
Facilitator	Enabler
Hardworking	Lazy
Kind	Cold

EMOTIONAL TRIGGERS FOR EARTH

HAPPY: Starting organizations

Making money

Steak dinners

Physical contact

ANGER: Upsetting their routine

Impractical ideas

Talking not doing

Pesky setbacks

FEAR: Lack of stability

Being poor

Changes

Lack of control

SAD: Unfinished business

Lack of routine

Being ill

Dishonesty

EXERCISE TRAITS FOR EARTH

Prefers warm up before/after workouts

Likes routine in their exercise

Prefers outdoor exercise

Likes afternoon or evening workouts

Can exercise two times a day

Able to exercise alone or in a group

Likes to cross-train

Superb endurance

Loves to stretch

Can combine water/ground exercises

SUGGESTED EXERCISE
FOR EARTH

Distance walking

Cross country skiing

Martial Arts

Bodybuilding

Triathlons/Ironman

Marathons/Ultramarathons

Distance swimming

Rowing

Roller blading

Distance cycling/ElliptiGo

WATER ELEMENT

"Try to be a rainbow in someone's cloud." Maya Angelou[82]

Water Elements see life as a journey and each movement they make is poetry in motion to a definite path. Sometimes it can be an unexpected one. To say the least, they are the most mystical and psychic of all the four elements. Unlike the Earth Elements, they are more interested in the spiritual than the physical wellbeing.

---

[82] https://www.goodreads.com/quotes/103456-try-to-be-a-rainbow-in-someone-s-cloud

"The spirit is larger than the body. The body is pathetic compared to what we have inside us." Diana Nyad[83]

Water is as dense as solid matter, but it responds readily to the slightest touch or a breeze and so it goes with those of the Water Element. Their feelings can fluctuate on a dime but they are gifted with a colorful and insightful imagination.

"Nothing is impossible. With so many people saying it couldn't be done, all it takes is

---

[83] https://www.azquotes.com/quote/835290

imagination." Michael Phelps[84]

They become submerged in their surroundings and can sense hidden emotional imbalance in any given situation.

Water Elements are shaped by their relationships with others. They love to be close to family and friends, but also need the restoring space of solitude to give them their inner peace.

Still waters run deep with Water Elements as they tend to keep their innermost feelings to themselves. This element type doesn't hold a grudge, but it will remember each

---

[84]https://quotefancy.com

detail of an event, good or bad.

As the Fire Elements are inclined to live in the present and rarely revisit their past, Water Elements are the opposite. They love to reminisce about the past. Since these tender souls are the most emotional of all the four elements, they embrace their cherished memories. Water Elements reflect on old times and look up old family and friends no matter what.

Their beloved past can have a powerful and positive impact on their present as well as leading them to a blissful future.

"If we open a quarrel between past and present, we shall find that we have lost the future." Winston Churchill [85]

Being an ultrasensitive element, their feelings can be hurt easily, so they are very protective of their delicate feelings in any given situation. This element can use exercise to meditate, to help soothe and nurture their delicate feelings, as well as protect themselves from being hurt.

"Swimming is probably the ultimate of burnout sports. It's

---

[85] quotationspage.com/quote/41666.html

ironic because millions of people who swim as their regular exercise love the meditation aspect of it; you don't wind up with any orthopedic injuries." Diana Nayad[86]

Compassion and caretaking are at the top of their list. The Air Elements are concerned with justice for all, but the Water Elements are devoted to healing all. However, they can be just as satisfied with helping people one at a time, especially those closest to their hearts. Nurturing gives them

---

[86]https://quotesgram.com/thomas-from-maze-runner-quotes

an inner peace and satisfaction to the extent of putting others before themselves.

These resourceful, yet sympathetic dreamers are associated with the color of blue and white and embrace the flowing movement that water or ice imbues them with. They cherish their alone time, so they don't become overwhelmed by emotional debris, which will disconnect them from their natural gift of intuition.

"Swimming is normal for me, I'm relaxed, I'm comfortable, and I know my surroundings. It's my home." Michael

Phelps.[87]

Their artistic endeavors are essential with helping them to express their inner thoughts and emotions as well as to release them from their own passing dramas.

Many metaphysicians declare water as the most powerful of all the elements because of its adaptability. It is clever and can work its way around or through any obstacle. The Water Element prefers to be in its own terrain, whether it be in water or on ice moving with a physical expression

---

[87] https://www.brainyquote.com/quotes/michael_phelps_167148

of freedom.

"For me, personally, skiing holds everything. I used to race cars, but skiing is a step beyond that. It removes the machinery and puts you one step closer to the elements. And it is a complete physical expression of freedom." Robert Redford[88]

Another client of mine, Ms. Lyn, said she was always too busy to exercise. She worked a fulltime job, visited her aunt in a nursing home, and took care of her ninety-three-

---

[88]https://unofficialnetworks.com/2015/08/11/top-10-ski-quotes-by-famous-personalities/

year old mother at home. At the same time, she was trying to deal with a bout of cancer. (At least those were the excuses she whispered to herself.)

Food comforted her, but she was not feeling healthy or fit by being overweight. When I told her about the book I was writing, she became interested in how it worked. We went through the quiz and found she was a Water Element.

One of the things she liked doing was getting on ancestry.com to look for information about her past relatives. She ended up with a big spread sheet of names and was able to reach back five generations.

It didn't surprise me that she was a Water Element. All the signs were there; caretaking, taking a personal interest in her family tree, and to top it off, she read tarot cards. I invited her to swim with me in the pool, and she swam like a mermaid. It's one of the exercises that Water Elements love to do.

We figured out a way for her to squeeze in a swimming workout almost every day, and she continued to take short walks with her dogs. Her food cravings began to dwindle, and she soon began seeing her weight drop.

Today Ms. Lyn looks forward to

getting in the water and added a belly dance class to her exercise routine.

PERSONALITY TRAITS FOR WATER

<u>POSITIVE</u>	<u>NEGATIVE</u>
Sympathetic	Cold
Sensitive	Indifferent
Sentimental	Cynical
Creative	Blocked
Cautious	Careless
Friendly	Distant
Compassionate	Harsh
Intuitive	Calculating
Listener	Talkative
Observant	Inattentive

EMOTIONAL TRIGGERS FOR WATER

HAPPY: People that text first

Long hugs

Listening to others

Being creative

ANGER: Unsolved issues

Being bullied

Being abandoned

Being taken for granted

FEAR: Being overly sensitive

Not feeling needed

Emotional loss

Being vulnerable

SAD: Losing family member

Harshly confronted

Hurt feelings

Being overly sensitive

EXERCISE TRAITS FOR WATER

Performs well in groups

Creative with exercise

Likes to be coached

Prefers afternoon workouts

Likes to meditate

Workout with a partner

Prefers outdoors

Likes the ice

Adores the water

Loves to stretch

SUGGESTED EXERCISES FOR WATER

Swimming

Water Polo

Surfing

Scuba Diving

Snowboarding

Ice Skating

Skiing

Synchronized Swimming

Yoga

Creative Dance

Synchronized Diving

SUMMARY OF THE FOUR ELEMENTS

Congratulations! Now that you know your element type, you can re-read that portion and become more familiar with your element. The following is a re-cap of all the element types.

If you are a **FIRE ELEMENT,** you are best described as a person of action. You get things done fast and never seem to wind down, like the Energizer Bunny. You are spontaneous and daring, living in the precious present, but are excited about what the future holds for you.

You'll fancy exercises that help expel all that energy you have inside. There are specific exercises for Fire, but it is the only element that can do it all. This element is fearless and is willing to try anything.

Therefore, your choice of exercises would be ones that are quick with short bursts. You'll like being out of your comfort zone with action and surprise. You need speed! You need to be on the go. You'll like sprints, racquetball, tap dancing, and Zumba…anything staccato and challenging.

The **AIR ELEMENTS** tend

to be inquisitive and innovative, living in the future. You are always in a fervent search for the new and different.

You prefer middle to long distance workouts, slowly building up speed to get into your groove. Playing golf, walking, cycling or jogging outdoors is right up your alley.

The treadmill would also suit you because you can choose the time, distance and dynamics of your workout. In fact, most of the gym equipment, like the elliptical, cycling, and the stair master, would fit the bill. You always relish trying something new. Check out the new

Gyro tonic method of exercise.

An **EARTH ELEMENT** is powerful and determined. You feel past events affect your future outcome, and you are committed to finishing what you start.

Distance is a natural for you but be sure to build up your endurance first. Determination is on your side to accomplish anything you put your mind to.

A triathlon or marathon is right up your alley, so you might want to try using the 'ElliptiGo' to help you train…it's easier on the joints. If you're not inclined to take on such endeavors, look at bodybuilding or martial arts.

WATER ELEMENTS will be drawn to do something pertaining to the good old H_2O; "in" the water, like swimming, or on the ice, like skiing. Water attracts you whether it's frozen or wet.

Be careful not to hang onto past events for a lengthy period-of-time, because it prevents you from forging ahead with your life. You'll enjoy scuba diving, swimming, synchronized swimming, and surfing. The gracefulness and finesse of these types of exercises will fit your artistic flare.

Don't forget you also need to get your feet on the ground at some point…so ice skating, snowboarding or some type of creative dance would also be good choices; even a good old snowball fight! Have fun!

CONCLUSION

***"Success is liking yourself, liking what you do, and liking how you do it." Maya Angelou.*[89]**

Kudos! Now you have actively experienced how to find your element: Fire, Air, Earth or Water. You have accomplished the essence of this exercise by identifying with one of the four element's characteristics that matches your exclusive psychological makeup. Every one

---

[89]https://www.goodreads.com/quotes/1208-success-is-liking-yourself-liking-what-you-do-and-liking

of you is different, and the suggested exercise traits and exercises in this book, are listed for your specific element type.

Doing one or more of these exercises will keep you fit through the power of your element, and you won't have to be consumed with counting calories. Why? Because you are engaging in the right exercise.

Finding your true element is your ticket to being fit physically, emotionally, and spiritually. Exercising will simply become a habit that you choose to perform in your life and will rid yourself of any emotional eating. Take the information you have just read and put your wheels and mind in motion.

A reminder: Don't be fooled and buy what fitness moguls profess. A one-size-fits-all has no room in the process of being fit whether it's exercise or diet.

I have accomplished my goal of inspiring people to do the very things they thought they couldn't do. Seeing their successes by using my "Bonnie Theory" has been awesome.

Whether you are young or old, male or female, this book is designed to work for you. Remember, your body and mind are the only ones you have.

Finding the right exercise played

a significant role in changing my outlook on life and put me in the best physical shape I have ever been in and continues to do so. It changed me from "Bonster the Monster" into "Inspirational Bonnie". Now let's see how enjoying exercise will make a change in your life.

I hope this journey of learning how to pick the right exercise, per your unique element, has been an enlightened one. You can now take control of your life and seize the vitality you were meant to enjoy. There is nothing like the present moment to begin a fit life.

"The way to get started is to quit talking and start doing."
Walt Disney[90]

---

[90]https://philosiblog.com/2012/06/22/the-way-to-get-started-is-to-quit-talking-and-begin-doing/

FINDING THE RIGHT EXERCISE

www.ingramcontent.com/pod-product-compliance
Lightning Source LLC
Chambersburg PA
CBHW050906260726

48660CB00001B/62